DEPARTMENT OF HEALTH AND SOCIAL SECURITY

Priorities in the Health and Social Services

The Way Forward

Further discussion of the Government's national strategy based on the consultative document Priorities for Health and Personal Social Services in England

September 1977

London: Her Majesty's Stationery Office

ISBN 0 11 320676 3

Contents

Foreword

In March 1976 my predecessor published a consultative document on priorities in the health and personal social services. This opened up a public debate to which many have contributed. I wish to thank all those who have sent in their comments and criticisms. The document was also used by health authorities in their strategic planning.

Now this new document continues the debate; it certainly does not conclude it.

There has been little criticism of the long-term aims set out in the consultative document. But considerable doubt has been expressed on whether it is practicable to achieve them within the suggested time scale. While the Government has ensured that there will continue to be at least a modest rate of increase in resources for these services in the country as a whole, I appreciate that we cannot hope to make significant and rapid changes in the desired directions without a more rapid growth of resources. On the one hand, we need to channel extra resources to those parts of the country with greater than average health needs which have been poorly provided for in the past. On the other hand we need to improve the care of children, the elderly, the mentally ill, the mentally handicapped and the physically handicapped as well as to finance important new developments in therapy. A more rapid rate of growth, both of revenue and capital resources, must depend on an improvement in the general economic situation. I hope we shall not have to wait too long.

It is not only the limited rate of growth of revenue which prevents us making rapid change. Much of what can be done is conditioned by what has already been achieved. New buildings may need to be provided and professional skills redeployed. Plans (particularly those involving major buildings) launched several years ago are coming to fruition and we must make the best possible use of them. Inevitably the capacity for change varies in different parts of the service and in different parts of the country.

In view of all these constraints, it would be easy for us to postpone the effort involved in moving to new priorities until the impact of past plans has been absorbed and until it is possible to provide a more rapid growth of resources. But this would be wrong. We must be clear about the road we are all trying to take even though our progress will be uneven. National policies must be clearly stated. The public, the authorities, the professions and all who work in health and social services expect a clear lead from the Government on the way forward.

I am convinced that there is scope for making faster progress in the desired directions by making better use of the resources which we have already. During the last few months I have travelled all over the country, talking to people in the health service about the way they do their work.

I have been greatly encouraged by the ingenuity they have shown in finding ways of using resources more effectively. I have added a note to this document which sets out some of the ideas which have been put to me. It is far from being a complete list, but it does suggest ways in which we could use the over £5 billion spent on the NHS to even better advantage.

Despite the immediate difficulties, we must be clear on what we want to achieve — on what our services should look like in the future when we can afford to provide them. The challenge is to give the public the very best services we can out of the money they are paying for them.

David Ennals.

1   The Broad Approach

1.1   The setting of priorities is not new; the challenge is to implement them. Part of the challenge — acceptance of the changes that must take place — is being met already by those who work in the National Health Service and the personal social services. But it is vital also that the public accept the changes. This is the other important part of the challenge which requires all our efforts.

Public expectations of the health and social services will frequently outrun supply and sometimes hard decisions will be needed to hold back some services to allow others to be developed. Here Community Health Councils (CHCs) have a key role in influencing public expectations and in helping health authorities to achieve a better use of resources.

To redistribute resources geographically, so reducing the disparity in health provision in different parts of the country, is the object of the methods established by *Sharing resources for health in England* (the Resource Allocation Working Party (RAWP) report). This is an important priority but it creates its own difficulties; some will think the pace too fast, others too slow.

To achieve a national pattern based on national priorities means redistributing real resources, money and manpower, between the main services. This can only happen to the best public benefit if health and social services professions play a full part through planning and joint planning systems, with all staff being involved in matters which affect them.

1.2   In setting priorities for the NHS and the personal social services, not only the links between these two services must be recognised but also the basic differences in their organisation and accountability. The legislation affecting the local authority social services imposes mandatory duties and confers substantial powers, but it also leaves scope for local variations in the extent and nature of services and how they may be provided; local authorities are accountable to their own electorate.

1.3   The first step toward a national pattern was taken with the publication in 1976 of the consultative document *Priorities for the health and personal social services in England*. This set priorities against the resources planned to be available in the years 1975/76 to 1979/80, outlining the strategy for the next decade. And this broad outline still stands as the basis upon which the Government are working.

1.4   This new document is complementary to, and should be read with the consultative document for it does not repeat detail nor follow the same presentation. It reports the comments received in response to the first document and concentrates on where changes and clarification are required. It reflects consultations over the past year, developments in the economic situation, and policy decisions — such as the RAWP report — which have intervened. It continues the debate which is to become a regular exchange between central and local government, the health authorities, the professions and the staff providing these services, and the public.

1.5   The pattern and pace of development of priority services will depend very much on the better use of resources overall, a point that cannot be over-emphasised. Here the general direction of service development is described but not the pace of change; all localities are different in terms of their present baseline, the relationship between their resources and measured need, their ability to achieve change, and the long-term requirements of their population. Some figures are given which are comparable to those in the consultative document but they illustrate only a *broad national picture* based on the assumptions that have been made; they are *not specific targets* to be reached by declared dates in any locality. They indicate the *national* long-term direction of strategic development within resource constraints, representing the best analysis that can be made nationally of the priorities Ministers wish to move towards. See Appendix VI: Background note.

PUBLIC EXPENDITURE SURVEY

1.6   The consultative document was based on the 1975 public expenditure decisions (Cmnd 6393). Some changes were made in resource assumptions in 1976 (Cmnd 6721); in particular, some reduction in capital for both health and personal social services in 1977/78 and 1978/79; increased dental and ophthalmic charges; and measures to reduce drug costs. However, the Government has planned to allow resources for health and personal social services to increase over the next few years. See Appendix IV. For the NHS, the money available will be enough in principle to meet increased demand arising from demographic change and leave a very small margin for other demands on the service. Some increased resources will be available also to the local authorities, supplemented by steadily increasing contributions by health authorities to the cost of jointly planned social services activities. This will provide a sound base from which further expansion can take place when economic circumstances allow. But even if there were a swifter expansion, available resources would not meet all demands. The need to choose will always be present.

POPULATION PROJECTIONS

1.7   Population projections are vital to effective planning (Figure 1).

FIG. 1 Population changes (England) 1976 based projections

1976 = 100

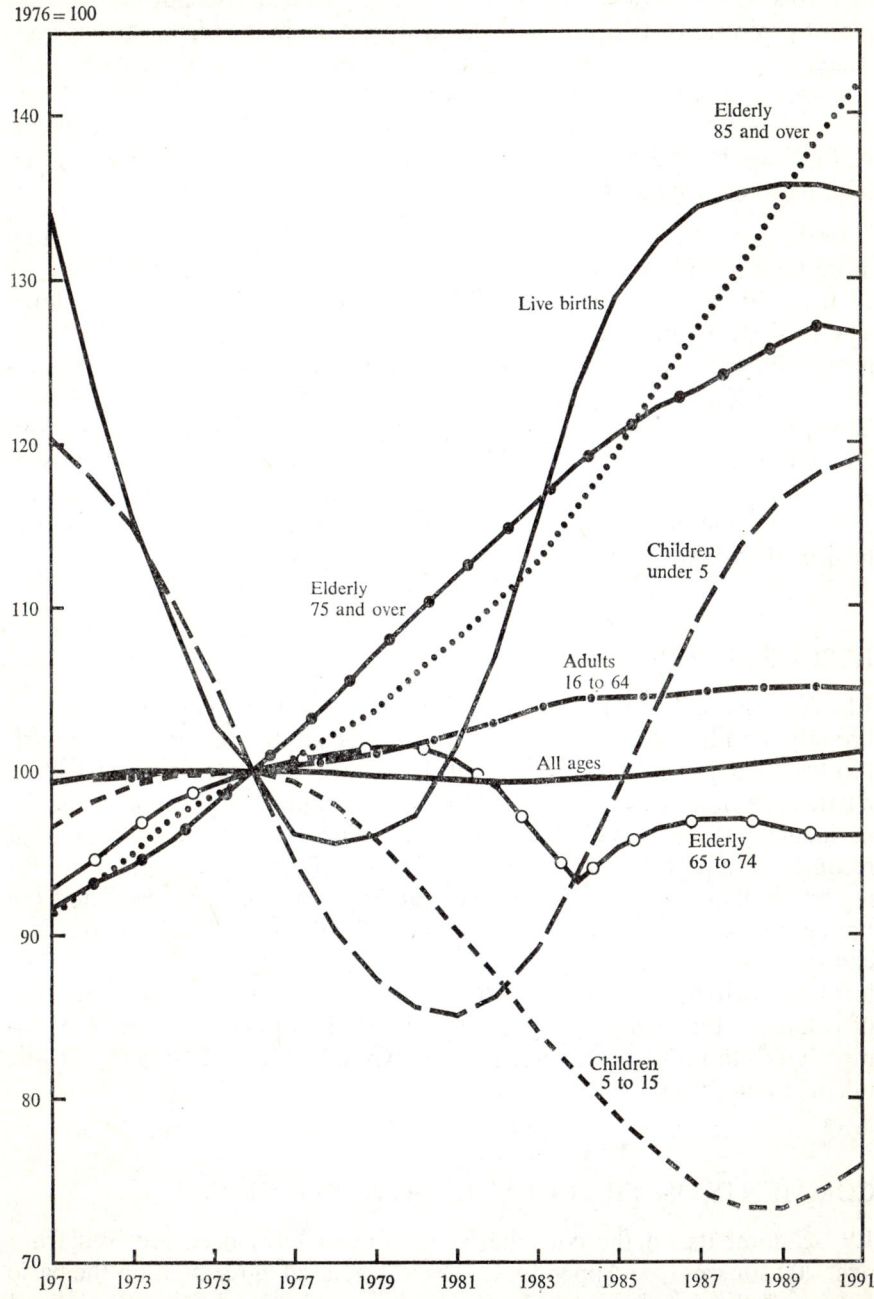

In recent years, projections of the number of births have indicated a continuing decline followed by a swift rise. The 1976 based projections of births again show a decline followed by a swift rise but, as with all recent projections, the timing of the upward turn in the birth rate has been delayed by a further year. The number of women of child-bearing age is known, but uncertainty remains as to the likely timing of births and size of families. This difficulty was recognised in the consultative document. Authorities should continue to use official "central" projections while taking proper account of local factors.

In the last 10 years the number of people aged over 65 has increased by more than a million. They now total more than $6\frac{1}{2}$ million, which is over 14 per cent of the population — and nearly a third of them live alone. The projections indicate a continuing increase in both the numbers and proportions of old people in the population with a particularly rapid increase projected in the number of people aged 75 and over. Over the next 20 years, the over 75s are expected to increase by nearly a third — from $2\frac{1}{3}$ million to just under 3 million. People aged over 85 are at present about one in a hundred of the population — and nearly half of those who are in the community live alone; by the year 2001 their proportion is projected to increase to about one in seventy-five.

RESOURCE PROJECTIONS

1.8   The process of gradual redistribution of resources is to be continued broadly in line with the principles established by the RAWP report, though their precise application will be refined over the years. It will be particularly important to redistribute within regions, in keeping with the national approach. The policies in this document rest on the long-term resource assumptions in Appendix V. The effect for particular health regions will depend on a variety of factors: some can be predicted (eg population changes); others are more difficult to forecast (eg possible changes in cross-boundary patient flows and in relative morbidity). For local authorities, account needs to be taken of the effect of redistribution of resources through rate support grant (RSG) settlements. The Government's White Paper on inner-city areas (Cmnd 6845) will also have to be taken into account.

COMMENTS ON THE CONSULTATIVE DOCUMENT

1.9   Comments on the consultative document have been received from over 200 sources (see Appendix I). There is general agreement on the basic nature of the problems and a recognition of the need for a disciplined approach to setting priorities. It is not possible to cover or to answer every point made but the main issues from the comments summarised in Appendix I are dealt with and other points will be taken into account in the further development of national policies.

1.10 Community Health Councils have been given a special role in relation to the planning process, in setting priorities and in encouraging a better use of resources. Their comments on the consultative document (on such issues as the use of voluntary effort to supplement resources, the particular problems of vulnerable sections of the community, and the need to cut out waste) show that they have recognised and accepted this responsibility.

RHA STRATEGIC PLANS

1.11 The first Regional Health Authority strategic plans have been received. At this very early stage of the NHS planning process most of the plans are necessarily tentative and incomplete. They will be revised for resubmission in January 1979. But they give a broad indication of the extent to which health authorities' plans follow national policies and priorities and the reasons for divergence from them, for example, because of special local circumstances, or financial or other constraints. Issues have been identified for discussion with individual regions, which may lead to some further adjustments to national policies and priorities. A detailed summary will be published after full discussion with all the RHAs. Some important general points have been derived from the first stages of the analysis (Appendix II), and these are reflected in subsequent chapters. (Figure 2 contains a regional analysis of expenditure per head of population by main programme).

1.12 The comments on the consultative document and the content of RHA strategic plans indicate clearly the impracticability of achieving *all* the identified priorities within the next 10 years. This is accepted. The pattern and pace of change will vary from place to place.

PLANNING OF LOCAL AUTHORITY SOCIAL SERVICES

1.13 Local authorities have developed their own systems of forward planning for personal social services, which have not been drawn together since local government reorganisation in 1974 to provide a national picture of the services with which they are concerned. As a start, they have been invited to submit information, by 1 October 1977, about their social services provision for the period 1976/77 to 1979/80. This return of local authority summary plans will be the first in an annual cycle and will be modified in the light of consultation and experience. The returns are designed to give an idea of the direction in which authorities propose to plan their services and so to help in setting assumptions for central planning.

FUTURE DEVELOPMENTS

1.14   The main aims remain broadly as follows:

to emphasise prevention;

to remedy past neglect of services, particularly those for the mentally ill and the mentally handicapped;

to make provision for the continuing increase in the elderly population and for the increasing number of children in local authority care.

EXISTING PRESSURES AND COMMITMENTS

1.15   There are however some formidable pressures on resources and a number of major commitments:

economic circumstances add to the pressures on families and communities for whom the health and social services must provide support and help;

geographic redistribution of health resources must continue;

training and education programmes for both health and personal social services must not be neglected;

revenue consequences of capital developments have to be met by both health and local authorities either at the expense of other developments or by savings through rationalisation or by reductions in other services; otherwise the commissioning of new facilities will need to be postponed;

relative gaps in services, particularly hospital acute services, and primary care facilities, especially in deprived areas, will have to be filled as soon as possible;

contractual costs arising from schemes in earlier capital programmes now abandoned or deferred will be a charge on current programmes.

1.16   These pressures and commitments are bound to restrict freedom of manoeuvre by health and local authorities in the foreseeable future. But the central challenge is to make more effective use of every £ that is spent in terms of actual benefits to people. This is particularly important in view of increasing demands on resources and projected increases in unit costs. It should be an important element in training and education programmes.

1.17   The main emphasis in this chapter has necessarily been on the short-term difficulties that authorities have to contend with. As the general economy improves in the longer term, the health and personal social services should gain their full benefit. This document sets the general pattern and direction of development; it is the pace of change which is affected by short-term difficulties.

FIG. 2 Current Expenditure Per Head by Programme and Region

Hospital and community health services 1975/76: £ November 1975 prices

Population Unit	General and acute	Primary Care	Elderly	Mental Illness	Mental Handicap	Children	Maternity	All Expenditure	
	Total Resident	Total Resident	65 and Over	Total Resident	Total Resident	Under 15's	Total Births	Total Resident	RAWP weighted and adjusted
Northern	32	1·4	51	8·4	3·2	8·0	300	61	59
Yorkshire	32	1·3	53	7·4	2·9	7·0*	300	61	61
Trent	26*	1·3	50	6·2	3·6	7·0*	290	53*	56*
E Anglia	31	1·0*	46	7·0	3·3	7·1	290	58	60
NW Thames	44†	1·9	43	9·3	4·1	9·9	350	76	78†
NE Thames	44†	2·3†	52	8·0	3·1	9·2	440†	78†	76
SE Thames	43	1·7	44	8·4	3·4	9·0	400	76	74
SW Thames	38	2·0	49	11·4†	6·9†	10·0†	320	77	71
Wessex	30	1·3	44	7·9	2·8*	7·9	260*	57	60
Oxford	30	1·7	64†	5·5*	3·1	8·3	380	59	71
S Western	29	1·3	41*	7·4	5·1	7·3	400	60	61
W Midlands	30	1·5	56	6·6	2·8*	8·2	320	58	60
Mersey	36	1·3	54	9·2	3·2	8·4	360	67	63
N Western	35	1·5	47	6·1	3·1	8·2	290	62	56*
ENGLAND	34	1·6	49	7·7	3·6	8·2	340	64	64

† = Highest
* = Lowest

See Appendix VI: Background Note.

2 The Priorities

PREVENTION

2.1 The Government has already published a consultative document *Prevention and Health: Everybody's Business,* the introductory paper to a series of discussion papers the first being *Reducing the Risk: Safer Pregnancy and Childbirth,* and the second, *Occupational Health Services,* scheduled for later in the year. Other topics to be covered over the next three or four years will include nutrition, alcoholism and heart disease. The first report of the Expenditure Committee of the House of Commons on Preventive Medicine has re-affirmed the importance of prevention and in response to it the Government will issue a White Paper. One of the main aims of the new initiative on prevention is to encourage individual members of the public to accept greater responsibility for their own health. Here CHCs have an important contribution to make.

2.2 Some services are predominantly concerned with prevention; for example, health education, the health visiting services, immunisation, genetic counselling, ante-natal care and screening for foetal abnormalities, fluoridation and chiropody. But most health services have a preventive role where they are concerned for example with early detection and treatment of disease to lessen its effects. Prevention forms an important part of the day-to-day activity of most of those working in the health and personal social services. The primary health care team has the essential role of giving specific advice to individuals on how to remain healthy; and of forestalling admission to hospital or residential care by warning against the development of unhealthy habits or detecting early signs of disease.

2.3 **Health Education** The Expenditure Committee Report stressed the importance of health education and the need for more Health Education Officers. The Health Education Council are subsidising the training of suitable officers, and part of a £1m additional allocation to the Council will be used for this purpose. The number of Health Education Officers has increased but there is a need for still more to be appointed.

2.4 **Vaccination and Immunisation** The Government has endorsed the report of the Joint Committee on Vaccination and Immunisation which emphasises the benefits derived from immunisation and vaccination programmes. They look for an early increase in the rate of take-up from its undesirably low level, and every effort should be made to encourage this. Tracing contacts of notifiable diseases (now extended to cover Lassa Fever, Viral Haemorrhagic Fever, Marburg Disease, Rabies and other exotic diseases) and vaccination and treatment are expensive but inevitable.

2.5 Family Planning Services The benefits from a reduction in the number of unplanned pregnancies fully justify the cost of family planning services. But there is evidence that many people receiving domiciliary service are able and willing to visit a family planning clinic or general practitioner. All existing domiciliary provision should therefore be reviewed and its need questioned. Health authorities will in future be responsible for ensuring adequate training for staff engaged in family planning services, a commitment formerly met from central funds.

2.6 Social Services Almost all the work of the local authority and voluntary social services has a preventive element; this is not only in their work with children, where local authorities have a specific statutory responsibility, but also in their work with mentally ill, mentally handicapped, physically handicapped and elderly people. This element is prominent in the field as well as domiciliary and day care services, but residential services also contribute by increasing provision for short-term admissions to give temporary relief to families caring for handicapped or disturbed relatives of any age.

COMMUNITY CARE

2.7 The consultative document emphasised the importance of adjusting the balance of care to provide greater support in the community. In this document, the term "community" covers a whole range of provision, including community hospitals, hostels, day hospitals, residential homes, day centres and domiciliary support. The term "community care" embraces primary health care and all the above services, whether provided by health authorities, local authorities, independent contractors, voluntary bodies, community self-help or family and friends.

2.8 The adjustment in the balance of care will be gradual and slow. It is clearly undesirable and often more expensive to admit or to keep in district general hospitals or long-stay hospitals old or mentally ill or mentally handicapped people, who could properly be looked after in the community. This will be avoided only if adequate progress can be made in developing community services, including community hospitals. Progress will vary from place to place depending on economic constraints, local choice and differences in the existing levels of provision. Where the pace is slow the hospital service should continue to make adequate provision.

2.9 Social Work Training The expenditure projections in the consultative document included an element specifically allocated to social work training in 1979/80. But developments in other services suggest that it is unlikely that local authorities will be able to expand social work training to the extent envisaged. Training remains an important priority. This was reflected in general guidance on the rate support grant (RSG) settlement for 1977/78 and a further £0·5m is being made available from central funds. Discussions are continuing with the local authority associations on the best way of securing the greatest progress in subsequent years.

2.10 **Field social work and domiciliary services** Comments on the consultative document pointed to the need for greater emphasis on field work and domiciliary services, in preference to residential care. This has been reflected in the £6m transfer from capital to revenue in 1977/78 and in the general guidance on the RSG settlement for 1977/78. Residential care will continue to consume a high proportion of resources, and additions will be necessary where major deficiencies exist or are likely to occur (eg in provision for mental illness and mental handicap). But in considering changes in expenditure levels, the protection of and, where possible, the increase in field work and domiciliary services are likely to remain the right general strategy. There will necessarily be differences in need between areas and in the state of development both of personal social services and other related services such as education and housing. However, taking the national picture for the next decade, the hope is for a slightly higher rate of growth of field work and domiciliary services than was envisaged in the consultative document.

2.11 **Voluntary bodies** Several voluntary organisations drew attention to their economic difficulties and their reliance on support from health and local authorities. Some felt that the way in which the statutory services were organised and delivered diminished or even precluded the contribution of volunteers and voluntary organisations. Voluntary effort provides a much needed addition to total resources. The Good Neighbour Campaign is an example of how partnership can be developed. The role of voluntary organisations and their relationship to the activities both of statutory bodies and of private individuals require more attention; the forthcoming report of the Wolfenden Committee on the role of voluntary organisations will provide an opportunity for review and discussion. Meanwhile, the voluntary organisations and the health and personal social services at national and local levels must plan and work together.

2.12 **Primary health care** The NHS (Vocational Training) Act 1976, when it is in force, will require prospective general medical practitioners to undertake three years' vocational training — two in hospital and one in general practice. Consultation is in hand on a timetable for implementing these provisions. The continuing development of primary health care teams, and the attachment of social workers to them, should be encouraged. More health visitors are needed to improve the preventive services to children, and more district nurses for the care of the elderly in the community. The increase in expenditure, proposed in the consultative document, of 6 per cent per annum *nationally* for more district nurses and health visitors is reaffirmed.

2.13 Drugs costs The BMA have joined in the consideration of publicity aimed at reducing the drugs bill (£450m in 1976) and establishing principles of prescribing to which doctors might attach greater weight. Ways of providing more information about prescribing patterns and about drugs and their preferred applications are being examined. The Government are consulting the profession on the possibility of recommendations to prescribing doctors about choice of treatment and quantities prescribed and about publicity aimed at reducing unreasonable expectations by members of the public. In addition to its intrinsic cost, hospital prescribing has a considerable influence on patterns of treatment in the community; both hospital drug and therapeutics committees and departments of clinical pharmacology are asked to contribute to the efficient use of drugs by clinicians. Promotional costs accepted under the Pharmaceutical Price Regulation Scheme have been reduced; the eventual saving will be about £16m a year.

2.14 Health centres Health centres should continue to be developed, according to the criteria set out in the consultative document which gave priority to health-deprived areas. To make the best use of available capital, health authorities have been given discretion to include other suitable projects in their programmes, including the adaptation of existing NHS premises for the purpose of developing the activity of the full primary health care teams in such areas. The Government are considering even greater flexibility in the application of health centre policy.

2.15 Community Hospitals The consultative document saw the strategy of the hospital services as involving (a) hospitals developed as district general hospitals (DGHs) or retained—and if necessary developed—as part of a DGH complex and (b) smaller hospitals fulfilling the function of community hospitals. This is broadly confirmed. To implement this strategy some measures of rationalisation are likely to be needed involving the closure or change of use of some hospitals, as well as developments. In view of financial restrictions, especially in the capital programme, development is likely to be slower than originally hoped.

2.16 Wherever local hospitals are retained and are not part of a DGH service, authorities should regard them as community hospitals. They broadly fulfil the main function of providing hospital services for patients who do not need the full specialist facilities of a DGH, and are often nearer their own homes. In future, therefore, any retained local hospital may be classified and managed as a community hospital except where all the patients are exclusively under the care of consultants, supported by junior hospital medical staff, and the hospital forms part of a DGH complex operating from several sites. (Fuller details, for the purpose of statistical returns, will be sent to authorities later.) When appropriate, and practicable, authorities should develop community hospitals to provide effectively, among other services, rehabilitation and continuing care of elderly patients, including elderly severely mentally infirm.

2.17 Detailed aspects of the previous guidance on community hospitals (HSC(IS)75) should not stand in the way of flexible and practical solutions agreed locally. For example, where a particular hospital is in part being used usefully and economically to provide surgery or radiological or other diagnostic services to a scale beyond that envisaged in the previous guidance, having regard to the level of provision presently available in the district as a whole, such use may be continued in addition to any extension of provision for the care of the elderly. Policies for admission and discharge, control of beds and clinical responsibility for patients need to be agreed between the authority on the one hand and consultants and general practitioners on the other after full local consultation.

SERVICES

2.18 The priorities for community care remain broadly as in the consultative document, with the following variations and adjustments:

Elderly people Because of the difficulties of increasing residential care for elderly people, the need for meals, home helps and chiropody services will be greater than that suggested in the consultative document. Research is being carried out at York University into the costs of alternative patterns of care.

Physically handicapped people No changes are proposed in the priorities set out in the consultative document. But particular attention needs to be paid to the requirements of the Chronically Sick and Disabled Persons Act, notably section 2, the application of which should determine the level of expenditure on aids, adaptations, telephones and holidays. These services can make a crucial difference to whether a disabled person can remain at home. The reduction in the PSS capital programme will reduce the scope for priority additional purpose-built accommodation for the younger disabled. It will be all the more important that there should be close co-operation between the social service housing and health authorities in order to make the best use of available accommodation and to continue the process of reduction in the small number of younger disabled who are unsuitably placed in accommodation for the elderly. Encouraging progress is being made in providing housing suitable for disabled people. Comments on the consultative paper (Department of Environment, DHSS and Welsh Office) on responsibility for adaptations are being considered and definitive guidance will be issued shortly. A start is to be made in the near future with a pilot scheme for young people who are both deaf and blind.

Mentally ill and mentally handicapped people The latest statistics have shown a need to change the base and projections in the consultative document for local authority residential places and day care places (including adult training centres) for mentally ill and mentally handicapped people (Figure 5). The mentally handicapped group aged 16–25 should receive special attention. The ratio now suggested for residential places in the short term is one for a mentally handicapped child to every five for adults, compared with one to every six envisaged as the ultimate target in the White Paper (Cmnd 4683).

Children Comments received on the recommendations contained in the Court Report on Child Health Services are being studied and the Government expect to announce their views later this year. The development of the less formal approach to residential and day care for children and the increase in intermediate treatment schemes on the lines of the consultative document is strongly supported. Plans for the provision of additional residential accommodation have been scaled down, though standards of care must be maintained. There remains, however, an urgent need to increase the stock of secure accommodation.

HOSPITAL SERVICES

2.19 **Acute Services** To enable priority needs to be met, there has to be rationalisation and pursuit of economy in the acute sector, by releasing under-used or less well-used resources. This aspect of the strategy, spelt out in the consultative document, gave rise to more concern than any other. The requirement to restrain the growth of expenditure on acute services nonetheless remains. But the Government recognise the importance of the acute sector in meeting the needs of priority groups, particularly elderly people. There can be no general formula for achieving the necessary degree of economy nationally upon which the rest of the national strategy depends, but discussion of regional strategic plans against the background identified later in this document should enable agreement to be reached on the broad approach to be followed in each region. It is clear that circumstances and timescales will differ both between and within regions.

2.20 **Maternity and Care of the Newborn** England still lags behind many European countries, as the Court Committee pointed out, though infant and neo-natal mortality rates fell sharply in 1976. The differences between the best and worst areas, and the much higher rates in Social Classes IV and V, are particularly disturbing. It is important to seek to achieve a further reduction of the mortality rates. Concentration of provision in properly equipped and staffed units is likely to lead to improved standards of care for the newborn. This does not necessarily require more special care baby cots (except where there is clearly a shortage), but it does require better equipped units with enough staff with relevant training. Intensive care should be concentrated in a small number of regionally designated units. The proposition in the consultative document remains valid — that health authorities should save expenditure by identifying under-used and inefficient maternity units which may be closed where better alternative services exist. Health authorities should ensure that there is an adequate midwifery service working in the community as well as in hospitals to provide high standards of maternity care, especially for mothers who are discharged early from hospital.

2.21 **Elderly People**   The consultative document reviewed demographic changes and estimated that a number of additional beds would be needed to match the increase in the numbers of elderly people. But it is not only beds that are needed: it is the additional staff time and effort required to enable elderly patients to return home as quickly as possible. The appointment of additional medical, nursing or rehabilitation staff, with skill in caring for the elderly may be a better investment than providing more beds with existing staff. It is likely that a higher rate of patients treated can be secured by all disciplines which deal with the acutely ill elderly and that the additional number of beds needed in England will be significantly lower than the total proposed in the consultative document. Health authorities should examine the scope for providing these beds by re-assignment, bearing in mind continued pressure on all those specialties which deal with elderly people. Elderly patients should normally be accommodated in such a way that the best use is made of facilities for rehabilitation and authorities should ensure that as much emphasis as possible is placed on this aspect of care, and on the liaison arrangements between different disciplines necessary to secure it.

2.22   The policies for the other priority groups remain broadly as in the consultative document:

a.   **Physically handicapped people**   Health authorities should avert the build-up of excessively long waiting lists at centres providing the new head-worn hearing aid. Planning has begun of the new spinal injuries unit for the South of England.

b.   **Mentally handicapped people**   The 1969 minimum standards of staffing and facilities should be met and, where possible, exceeded.

c.   **Mentally ill people**   The release of really substantial resources for deployment on the development of local psychiatric services generally is likely to be achieved only with the closure of a whole hospital. Regions ought to be looking to the future and planning the replacement of major mental illness hospitals. It is important that in-patient and day hospital provision should be made locally for the elderly severely mentally infirm, using wherever possible suitable small hospitals no longer required for other purposes. In the meantime, adequate provision for such patients should continue in mental illness hospitals. Funds allocated for regional secure units should not be committed to other purposes, except on a strictly temporary basis.

d.   **Children**   There has been only limited progress with the rationalisation of children's hospital services. Bed occupancies are low in many children's wards: where this is because children are being nursed in adult

14

wards, they should be moved into children's departments as soon as possible: where low occupancy continues, there is likely to be scope for reducing the number of children's beds. The development of more day-patient and out-patient care for children will further reduce the need for expensive in-patient facilities. Handicapped children need multi-disciplinary assessment. There should be more paediatric dialysis.

ILLUSTRATIVE FIGURES

2.23 The consultative document contained tables and figures setting the priorities against the resources available in the form of a programme budget. Figure 3 compares the actual out-turn of expenditure for 1975/76 against the provisional estimate in the consultative document and includes a revised illustrative projection for 1979/80 on the basis of the revised priorities outlined above. It must be emphasised that the details in Figure 3 simply provide illustrative indications of the *national* long-term direction of strategic development within resource constraints; they do not represent specific targets to be achieved by declared dates in any locality. They represent the best quantitative assessment that can be made *nationally* of the priorities Ministers wish to see pursued. See Appendix VI.

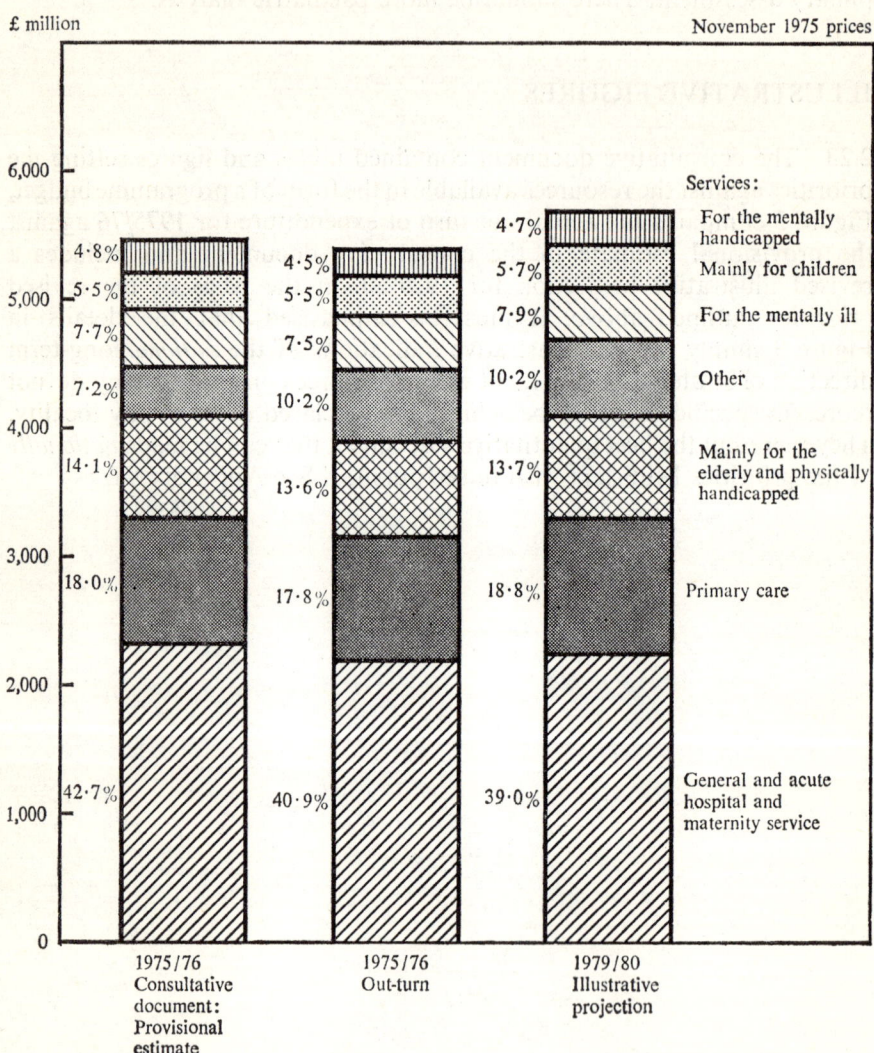

FIG. 3   **Health and Personal Social Services:**
Programme Expenditure as a percentage of total
(current and capital)

£ million   November 1975 prices

Services:

6,000

5,000

4,000

3,000

2,000

1,000

0

1975/76 Consultative document: Provisional estimate	1975/76 Out-turn	1979/80 Illustrative projection

4·8% / 4·5% / 4·7%   For the mentally handicapped
5·5% / 5·5% / 5·7%   Mainly for children
7·7% / 7·5% / 7·9%   For the mentally ill
7·2% / 10·2% / 10·2%   Other
14·1% / 13·6% / 13·7%   Mainly for the elderly and physically handicapped
18·0% / 17·8% / 18·8%   Primary care
42·7% / 40·9% / 39·0%   General and acute hospital and maternity service

This figure gives programme shares in the same format as Fig. 1 of the consultative document, but because of the change in the accounts the figures are not precisely comparable. See Appendix VI.

3   The Way Forward

3.1   Can it all be done? Many of those who commented on the consultative document doubted whether it had taken adequate account of the practical difficulties encountered in operating the services. Particular concern was also expressed about the extent to which plans for service development might be frustrated by unexpected calls on resources; this is an important point, and in drawing up the revised priorities some account has been taken of probable increases in unit costs because of such developments. See Appendix VI.

PRACTICAL CONSTRAINTS

3.2   Ministers acknowledge the practical difficulties with which authorities and staff will have to contend in planning and operating services:

Regional Health Authorities (RHAs) have to cope with increased demands and new problems with little or no increase in resources. They also have to cope with the problem of redistributing existing resources to their own relatively deprived areas. This is particularly severe in the above target regions; but all regions are faced with the problems inherent in redistribution of resources.

Local authorities face similar problems, with limited resources and the redistributive effect of RSG settlements.

Authorities will sometimes need to spend in the short term in order to achieve savings for the longer term.

Re-deployment means services have to be rationalised and some facilities closed. This will often create difficulties with local interests.

A building which might be suitable for closure as part of an overall plan may have to be retained to provide a particular service even though, in some instances, it is not totally satisfactory for the purpose.

Capital developments to which an authority is already committed may have implications for resource use which effectively foreclose other desirable options for future planning.

These are real difficulties. They certainly affect the pace and opportunity for change; but they do not alter the objectives to which it is directed.

SERVICE DELIVERY

3.3   Health authorities are being asked to restrict the acute services in the NHS as a whole to a slower rate of growth than in recent years. This policy is adopted deliberately, with full awareness of the consequences which will vary according to local circumstances. In some districts, long-sought improvements will be further delayed. Some hospitals will have to continue to manage with facilities which are out-dated or inadequate. The expectations both of the professions and of users will not be fully satisfied. In other places where services are not under the same pressure, the provision of new facilities which are expensive will have to be postponed. This is the price which has to be paid if progress is to be made in those parts of the service which have been given priority for development. Much has already been done to increase the efficiency of acute services: the number of beds has been reduced by 4·6 per cent between 1970 and 1975 and the average length of stay shortened from 11·3 to 10·2 days. But the further restraint required implies increased rationalisation, closure of some units, curtailment of some services in some places and more effective use of staff and facilities generally.

3.4   Some authorities and professional bodies, individual doctors and nurses and others working in these services have warned of the frustration they will feel at continued delay in achieving their long-unfulfilled expectations. They are concerned that patients will suffer from real short-comings in these services. The extent to which actual short-comings in services can be reduced, and therefore the extent to which the professions can be encouraged to participate fully, will depend on:

first, the vigorous pursuit of efficiency and economy, not only in the acute services, but wherever in the health and personal social services resources could be better used;

second, recognition of the priority pressures *within* the acute services;

third, the willingness of those concerned, especially those in the professions, to accept the policy and to join in planning for it;

fourth, the skill with which the planning is done and the time scale for changes: planned measures tend to hurt less than hasty ones. It is not the intention of the Government to rush the acute services into sudden restraint.

3.5   At the same time health and local authorities have to cope with the demands presented by an increasing number of old people. This places increasing burdens on general practice and the community nursing services and on the personal social services — including day-care, home helps and meals services — and on residential care. But, equally important, it leads to increased demands by the elderly on almost every bit of the acute hospital services, with only a part of this acute care being provided by the hospital geriatric team. Given the high incidence of psychiatric illness in elderly people, a further burden is placed on the psychiatric services; and this in turn leads to an increased demand for long-stay care for those who prove incapable of managing outside hospital.

3.6   Ministers confirm the broad objectives in the consultative document. But a look at one facet of the changes proposed — increase in the geriatric hospital provision to be made possible only by restraining additional expenditure on acute hospital services — leads to the conclusion that:

> a steady rate of progress is not practicable nationally: redeployment and rationalisation of acute services requires careful planning and perhaps initially a substantially more rapid increase in expenditure than implied in the consultative document (to be offset in later years);
>
> what is not practicable nationally is even less practicable in some local areas.

This view is supported by the analysis of RHA strategic plans. For example, in an above target region it may be necessary to devote part of the capital programme to rationalising acute services before resources can be released for other priorities; in a below target region, the capital facilities coming on stream may dictate that gaps in acute services are made good first, leaving other deficiencies to be tackled later. The results may be that the expansion of, for instance, geriatric medicine has to be postponed, and this may also be held back by the shortage of geriatricians.

3.7   But these particular objectives can be shown to be achieved without so pronounced a swing in the balance of expenditure. The role of acute geriatric services is to achieve diagnosis, treatment, social assessment and rehabilitation of the elderly patient by skilled attention to his needs as an elderly person: rehabilitation may equally be achieved if the treatment provided to him under the care of the general physician, or orthopaedic or general surgeon, is similarly directed with advice, as appropriate and necessary, from the geriatric team. While the public record will not show this as a development in the acute geriatric services, the statistics for length of stay of elderly patients will, over time, reveal the extent to which rehabilitation is being achieved.

3.8   The general extent of the pressures that the acute services will face in view of the growing numbers of old people was stressed in comments on the consultative document. This is illustrated by the following table:

Average daily available beds used by elderly patients
Hospital In-patient Enquiry: 1974 (England and Wales)

Specialty	Aged 65–74		Aged 75 and over	
	Number of beds	% of beds	Number of beds	% of beds
All non-psychiatric	33,833	19	57,101	31
General Medicine	7,730	28	5,965	22
Geriatric Medicine	10,691	21	38,016	74
General Surgery	5,478	22	4,053	17
Orthopaedic Surgery	2,750	15	4,250	25

The pressure will, however, vary considerably in different areas and districts. Plans for the acute services should be framed to deal with expected local needs, drawing on experience of local patterns of provision (including different rates of development of community services). New guidance will be available from the DHSS during the coming year on long-term target bed/population ratios for the various acute disease categories. To assist consideration of services for the elderly centrally, the new programme budget projections have been based on separate consideration of geriatric care for the first three months following admission and of long-term care; the projections assume that the number of cases will grow at over 2 per cent per year but that this increase will be mainly short-stay, implying higher throughput and fewer beds per 1,000 elderly population (Figure 4). Health authorities should consider the adoption of a similar distinction to assist their local planning.

3.9   This points to the following main priorities within the acute sector:

concentrate acute services including those for the elderly in the newest and most suitable premises (closing if necessary less suitable facilities, and those which are unduly expensive to maintain);

direct capital in the short term to small schemes designed to assist rationalisation—especially closures—and to help avoid the further deterioration of known black spots (eg long waiting times);

encourage local initiatives to make the most effective use of nursing and remedial staff (short lengths of stay and numbers of increasingly frail elderly patients must add to the work of these professions);

develop day surgery, five day wards and programmed investigation units;

pursue the possibility of rationalising the provision of regional specialties (to ensure that there is maximum efficiency in the use of expensive facilities and that each unit has a sufficient load to maintain and develop standards).

3.10   But a number of pressures will be encountered, and authorities will meet others as their planning proceeds:

additional transport will be needed to cope with the increased provision of day care, including geriatric day hospitals;

improvements in the primary health care field will require additional work from hospital pathological and X-ray departments in support;

preventive aspects of obstetric care will need attention, including genetic counselling and pre-natal screening for foetal abnormality;

rehabilitation should have priority, either in the ward setting or in special units designated for this purpose; through improvements in remedial profession staffing; and generally as an aim of many more clinical teams;

long, unplanned waiting times for non-urgent admissions may cause higher human and resource costs which early admission might avoid in some cases. Local study may identify action to be taken which would help to avoid lengthening waiting times. Authorities should continue to set themselves target waiting times of not more than one month for urgent and twelve months for non-urgent treatment (HSC(IS)181).

MEDICAL MANPOWER

3.11 Because of delays in completing capital projects, it will not be possible to reach the target medical school intake of some 4,000 a year in 1980. But the Government continue to place high priority on the achievement of this target by the early 1980s, to enable a higher proportion of posts in hospitals and general practice to be filled by British graduates, and to help bridge the gaps in services. The priority of the medical training programme will however have to be sustained within available resources which will have to finance the new hospitals built partly to meet service needs but also to provide training facilities for doctors. This could cause some further delay in reaching the target. It is clearly important that sufficient pre-registration posts should be available for the increasing output of graduates, and that there should be full oportunity for postgraduate training. It remains essential for the NHS to make full use of available medical manpower, and to ensure that posts are available for doctors with domestic commitments who cannot devote full time to the exercise of their professional skills.

THE KEY — GOOD PLANNING

3.12 **DHSS planning** The Department has been operating a planning system covering health and personal social services since 1974. The particular technique used for relating policies and priorities to resources is the programme budget. (The consultative document contained a description and details of the programme budget.) A revised national programme budget analysis has been prepared taking account of the 1976-based population projections, differences between the 1975/76 out-turn and the 1975/76 consultative document estimate, and revised assumptions for unit costs. The projections have been translated into implied levels of provision which represent broad *national* objectives (Figures 4 and 5). These are *not* specific targets to be achieved by declared dates, even at a national aggregate level. The 1979/80 projections are intended only to *illustrate* what might be achieved given provisional resource constraints. The projections are not based on any detailed information about the intentions of authorities nor do they take account of the most recent work connected with the rate support grant on personal social services which suggests that social work and home help services are likely to grow less than the projections envisage. See Appendix VI: Background note.

3.13 **PSS planning** For the personal social services, planning procedures will need to fit in with the wider planning arrangements and decision-making processes of the local authorities concerned. Whereas in central government the health and personal social services are combined in a

FIG. 4
FIG. 4 Hospital and Community Health Services
Average levels of provision and current expenditure per head

Service	Population Base	Level of Provision (per 1,000 appropriate population)		
		Departmental Guidelines	1975/76 Out-turn	1979/80 Illustrative Projection
		Available Beds		
Acute Inpatients	Total	2·8	3·4	3·1
Acute Outpatients	Total	—	...	...
Obstetric Inpatients	All Births	—	37·6	32·8
Obstetric Outpatients	All Births	—	...	...
Geriatric Inpatients	65 yrs and over	10·0	8·5	8·4
Geriatric Outpatients	65 yrs and over	—	...	...
Younger Disabled Inpatients	15–64 years	—	0·04	0·06
Mental Handicap Inpatients	Total	0·68	1·2	1·1
Mental Handicap Outpatients	Total	—	...	...
Mental Illness Inpatients	Total	0·5 ⎫		
Elderly Severely Mentally Infirm Inpatients	65 yrs and over	2·5—3·0 ⎬	2·1	1·9
Mental Illness Outpatients	Total	—	...	...
		Places		
Non-psychiatric Day Patients	65 yrs and over	2·7	1·1	1·0
Mental Illness Day Patients	Total	0·65 ⎫		
Elderly Severely Mentally Infirm Day Patients	65 yrs and over	2·0—3·0 ⎬	0·29	0·36
Ambulances	Total	—	...	...
Other hospital	Total	—	...	...
		Staff (WTE)		
Health Visiting	Total	0·33	0·15	0·18
District Nursing	Total	0·40	0·25	0·32
Midwifery	All Births	—	...	...
Prevention	0–4 years	—	...	...
Chiropody	65 yrs and over	—	...	...
Family Planning	15–64 years	—	...	...
School Health	5–15 years	—	...	...
Other Community Health	Total	—	...	...
Administration	Tota	—	...	...

See Appendix VI   ... = Not applicable

Throughput		Cost per Unit of Provision		Expenditure per Head of Population	
1975/76 Out-turn	1979/80 Illustrative Projection	1975/76 Out-turn	1979/80 Illustrative Projection	1975/76 Out-turn	1979/80 Illustrative Projection
Cases per bed		Cases		£	£
		£	£		
24·3	28·2	315	318	25·7	27·5
...	...	...	...	6·6	7·0
32·8	37·5	217	201	267·1	248·0
...	...	...	...	35·3	39·6
3·6	3·8	1,120	1,160	34·0	36·6
...	...	...	...	0·20	0·22
Occupancy Rate		Occupied Beds			
79%	85%	4,370	4,730	0·15	0·23
92%	92%	3,340	3,810	3·6	3·8
...	...	...	...	0·004	0·004
87%	86%	3,810	4,700	7·1	7·6
...	...	...		0·35	0·37
		Places			
...	...	1,530	1,530	1·7	2·0
...	...	1,050	1,050	0·30	0·38
...	...	...	...	2·0	2·1
...	...	...	...	2·9	3·1
		Staff (WTE)			
...	...	6,000	6,000	0·88	1·1
...	...	6,000	6,000	1·5	1·9
...	...	...	...	41·5	43·9
...	...	...	...	3·5	4·9
...	...	...	...	1·7	1·9
...	...	...	...	0·37	0·43
...	...	...	...	5·8	6·0
...	...	...	...	1·1	1·1
...	...	...	...	3·8	3·7

— = No guideline   WTE = Whole time equivalent

FIG. 5 Local Authority Personal Social Services
Average level of provision and current expenditure per head

November 1975 Prices

Service	Population Base	Level of Provision (per 1,000 appropriate population) — Departmental Guidelines	Level of Provision — 1975/76 Out-turn	Level of Provision — 1979/80 Illustrative Projection	Occupancy Rate	Cost per occupied place, available place, meal or staff — 1975/76 £	Cost — 1979/80 £	Expenditure per head of population — 1975/76 £	Expenditure — 1979/80 £
Residential		Available Places				Occupied Place			
—Elderly	65 years and over	25·0	18·1	17·9	95%	1,210	1,290	20·8	21·9
—Younger Disabled	15–64 years	—	0·45	0·46	95%	1,210	1,290	0·52	0·56
—Mental Handicap–Adults	16 years and over	0·78	0·28	0·35	95%	1,240	1,310	0·33	0·44
—Mental Handicap–Children	0–15 years	0·44	0·17	0·24	86%	3,240	3,440	0·47	0·71
—Mental Illness	Total	0·19–0·30	0·10	0·12	90%	920	980	0·08	0·10
—Children	0–17 years	—	3·5	3·9	84%	3,340	3,730	9·7	12·1
Day Care						Available Place			
—Elderly	65 years and over	3·4	2·6	2·7	...	560	560	1·5	1·5
—Younger Disabled	15–64 years	1·5	0·59	0·63	...	560	560	0·33	0·36
—Mental Handicap	Total	0·60	0·77	0·97	...	720	740	0·56	0·72
—Mental Illness	Total		0·10	0·19	...	560	560	0·06	0·11
—Day Nurseries	0–4 years	—	8·3	10·8	...	1,010	1,010	8·4	10·9
Other Services		Staff (WTE)				Staff (WTE)			
—Home Helps	65 years and over	12·0	6·5	7·1	...	2,210	2,210	14·3	15·7
—Social Workers	Total	0·44	0·44	0·49	...	4,590	4,690	2·0	2·3
		Meals Per Week				Meal			
—Meals	65 years and over	200	119	132	...	0·34	0·34	2·1	2·3
—Boarding out	0–17 years	—	...	...	...	...	...	1·2	1·3
—Aids, Adaptations, etc.	Total	—	...	...	...	...	...	0·26	0·27
—Intermediate Treatment	5–17 years	—	...	...	...	...	...	0·08	0·17
—Other LA Services	Total	—	...	...	...	...	...	0·59	0·58
—Administration	Total	—	...	...	...	...	...	2·5	2·6

See Appendix VI

... = Not applicable   — = No guideline   WTE = Whole time equivalent

single department, the local authorities are separated in the field fr
health authorities but combined with, or closer to, the authorities r
sible for education, planning, housing and other matters of local concern.
Their work with children also puts them into a close relationship with the
courts and the probation service. The central responsibilities in relation to
these functions are distributed among a number of government departments. Corporate planning at local level has therefore concentrated on
those activities for which local authorities hold direct responsibility.

3.14 Co-operation at a local level will be particularly important with
education authorities on issues concerning the under-fives and the mentally
handicapped, on problems such as truancy, and on children at risk of
injury or personal breakdown; with housing authorities on matters concerning the care of the elderly, hostels and homes for mentally ill and
mentally handicapped people, and families in need of support; with the
the local social security office on all matters of income maintenance; and
with the courts on matters concerning the care of children. These are only
the outstanding items; local circumstances will offer many more opportunities for joint action. The most significant might well come from the influence
of the social services team on their colleagues responsible for other
functions of the authority, to carry out those functions in a manner that
will be helpful and sympathetic to the clients and potential clients of social
services departments. The scope for such influence is perhaps greatest in
town planning, in transport, in the education service and in the planning,
design and administration of local authority housing.

3.15 **NHS planning** For the NHS, a planning system has been in operation
since April 1976. It takes account of the different functions of different
levels of the service, and distinguishes between strategic planning and
shorter term operational planning. There must be a real commitment at all
levels to planning as a systematic approach to identifying needs, considering priorities, devising realistic ways of implementing those priorities and
consulting and involving those whose interests are affected. It is worth
emphasising the following points:

> planning requires regular reviews of all services and resources, not
> simply the deployment of new money;

> the RAWP report emphasised the importance of following through
> proposals for geographical redistribution of health resources effectively
> in the planning process;

> while total self-sufficiency in any area or district is not a necessary aim,
> major imbalances in opportunity for access to services within a region
> need to be corrected over time in the planning and allocation process;

> the planning process gives effect to one of the most important features
> of NHS reorganisation—the involvement of clinicians in management at
> all levels;

> consultation is a vital element in planning, particularly with staff
> interests and CHCs;

priority selection through planning helps to show how resources can be redeployed to meet changing patterns of need and to take advantage of changing medical technology;

the Government need to be able to draw on authorities' plans when developing national policies and priorities.

3.16 Joint planning The initiative of central government, in promoting joint planning and joint finance (HC(77)17/LAC(77)10) over administrative boundaries that have not always been easy to cross at local level, is intended to complement the development of corporate planning within authorities. Funds voted for the services for which the Secretary of State is responsible cannot be used for the direct support of other Departments' services. But the Government are committed to a joint approach to social policy as is evident from the numerous joint operations between Departments.

3.17 Considerable anxieties were expressed by local authorities about their freedom of choice in joint financing and about their control over the bill they might ultimately have to pay even despite the lengthening of the period of commitment by the health authorities, variations in the proportions borne by either authority at the outset, and the inclusion of local authority schemes already in the pipeline. The scheme has however met with an imaginative and vigorous response from authorities. It can be expected to continue to make a significant contribution to the development of services. This year it has been possible to take the matter a stage further by inviting local authorities to submit their proposals for expenditure over the next three years. Future arrangements for joint finance envisage that local authorities will be able to rely on continuing and increasing support from this source for their social services expenditure until other methods of financing activities of joint concern are seen to become available.

3.18 Estate management One of the most important resources in the NHS is the health service estate, including a considerable acreage of land and a large stock of buildings. With money for new building restricted, the existing estate must be used to the best effect; authorities must ensure that buildings really meet current needs; and land acquisition, use and disposal must be kept in balance through the land programme. It is important to keep buildings and engineering plant in a good state of repair and operational efficiency. Maintenance is not an optional activity, it is a vital function which ensures that services to patients are not interrupted because of failures in the building fabric or in engineering services. But land and buildings that no longer serve existing or foreseen needs should be transferred, if appropriate, to the social services or disposed of for other use. A revised version of the DHSS handbook containing procedures on NHS land transactions and disposal of surplus land has recently been issued. RHA chairmen have been asked to ensure that the need to review all NHS land holdings is fully appreciated, particularly in areas and districts.

3.19 **Community health councils** CHCs have been invited to make a strong contribution to planning and to assist in the consideration of policy options and determination of priorities. Members of some CHCs take part as members of planning teams drawing up proposals for consideration by authorities. CHCs have a dual role; they have to communicate both with the authority and with the consumer. To give advice, CHCs need some feedback from the public. But before the public can offer a sensible view, it needs to understand the problem. It is important that CHCs should continue to be informed about, and discuss publicly, the real issues facing the local health service management — the scope for change and the need to determine priorities. The delivery of some services — particularly those of preventive medicine — is more effective where the public participates with understanding: to help this happen is a vital role for the CHC.

3.20 **Better use of resources** Management costs are already controlled (HC(77)10). Within the expenditure of the NHS it is generally accepted that there is scope for achieving a more effective use of resources. It will take time and the willing efforts of clinicians, managers and staff to achieve this. Priority will be given in national and local research to projects concerned with better use of resources. Appendix III gives some examples of good practice ideas. They will not be applicable everywhere — some will already have been widely introduced. Some will produce savings; others will enable a better service to be given to patients without spending more money. Resources released in this way should wherever possible be used in the area where the savings are achieved. A more effective use of resources can help to ensure that the policies described in this document can be implemented more quickly.

APPENDIX I

Comments on the Consultative Document on Priorities and Index of Commentators

1 The general principles of the strategy proposed were widely endorsed and the attempt to state national priorities in the context of available resources was generally welcomed.

2 The question causing most concern (particularly among representatives of the medical profession) was the degree of restraint on further growth proposed for the general and acute hospital services.

3 There was some misunderstanding of the proposals for increasing geriatric beds which was seen by some as calling for an increase in long-stay provision.

4 There were objections to the proposed reductions in spending on maternity services, from professional organisations with a special interest, which to some extent indicated a misunderstanding of the consultative document proposals.

5 Local authorities in general and many health authorities questioned the financial realism of the consultative document, and local authorities challenged some of the particular assumptions underlying the calculations.

6 Some local and health authorities questioned the philosophy of shifting resources from institutions to the community, on grounds of cost/benefit and financial feasibility.

7 Some CHCs emphasised the need to maintain services for the economically active population despite the claims of the priority services; and they also doubted their ability to influence the development of community based services through the Family Practitioner Service.

8 Local authorities generally criticised the document for taking a mainly health service perspective and because it did not adequately recognise the corporate element of local authority planning, and the links with housing, education, employment and the courts.

9 Advisory and professional bodies generally endorsed the broad lines of the proposed strategy but questioned individual aspects of it, particularly the proposals for the acute hospital and maternity services.

10 There was general acceptance of the proposed continued development of health centres as an important element in primary care services. A number of issues were raised, however, concerning difficulties which some authorities face in pursuing this policy, and the need for careful consideration of the differing needs of, eg, inner urban areas as compared with rural areas.

11 Some professional bodies suggested a different approach to the organisation and funding of the NHS as an alternative strategy.

12 The Trades Union Congress endorsed the broad lines of the strategy but had particular points to make on individual aspects. They were especially concerned about the substantial difference according to social class suggested by various health indicators*. Another point to which they attached particular importance was the need for greater emphasis on health education.

13 NHS staff bodies criticised what they saw as the low level of funding for the services and called for effective consultation with staff interests on the implementation of any strategy involving their future, but welcomed the CD's assurances that there were unlikely to be problems of manpower supply or redundancy and that training programmes would be maintained.

14 The voluntary bodies welcomed the document and endorsed the strategy, had particular points to make about individual aspects and emphasised the need for corporate planning — especially with housing, education and the environment — both centrally and locally.

---

*A Working Group on Inequalities in Health has been appointed under the Chairmanship of the DHSS Chief Scientist. The Working Group are examining the evidence on the relationship of health standards to social class, with a view to commissioning research.

Index of Commentators

HEALTH AUTHORITIES AND BOARDS OF GOVERNORS

National Association of Health Authorities

12 Regional Health Authorities

24 Area Health Authorities

Society of FPCs and 3 individual committees

Hospital for Sick Children
Royal National Orthopædic Hospital
Royal National Throat Nose and Ear Hospital

LOCAL AUTHORITIES

Association of County Councils
Association of District Councils
Association of Metropolitan Authorities
and 12 individual Local Authorities

COMMUNITY HEALTH COUNCILS

45 CHCs

PROFESSIONAL ORGANISATIONS AND ADVISORY BODIES

Association of Anæsthetists of GB & NI
Association of British Pædiatric Nurses
Association of Chief Administrators of Health Authorities
Association of Directors of Social Services
Association of Domestic Management
Association of Nurse Administrators
Association of Sterile Supply Administrators
Association of Supervisors of Midwives
Berkshire Local Medical Committee
British Association of Occupational Therapists
British Association for the Study of Community Dentistry
British Association of Social Workers
British Dental Association
British Dental Hygienists Association
British Dietetic Association
British Geriatrics Society
British Hospital Doctors Federation
British Medical Association
British Orthoptic Society
British Pædiatrics Association
Central Health Services Council
Central Midwives Board
Chartered Society of Physiotherapy
College of Speech Therapists
Committee of Vice Chancellors and Principals
Council for Postgraduate Medical Education in England
Council for Professions Supplementary to Medicine
Council for the Education and Training of Health Visitors
Croydon Area Chemists Contractors Committee
Cuckfield and Crawley District Medical Committee
Derbyshire Local Medical Committee
Faculty of Anæsthetists
Faculty of Community Medicine

30

Federation of Associations of Clinical Professors
Federation of Optical Corporate Bodies
General Medical Services Committee
General Nursing Council
Guild of Health Education Officers
Hertfordshire Branch of the Royal College of Midwives
Health Visitors Association
Hospital Caterers Association
Institute of Health Education
Institute of Home Help Organisers
Joint Committee of Ophthalmic Opticians
Joint Consultants Committee
Kensington Chelsea & Westminster Area Medical Committee
Kent Area Medical Committee
Leeds Joint Committee of Physicians
Leeds Western District Faculty
Medical Women's Federation
Merton Sutton and Wandsworth Local Pharmaceutical Committee
National Association of Theatre Nurses
National Development Group for the Mentally Handicapped
North Yorkshire Area Medical Committee
Panel of Assessors for District Nurse Training
Personal Social Services Council
Pharmaceutical Committee for South West London & Surrey
Pharmaceutical Services Negotiating Committee
Pharmaceutical Society of Great Britain
Residential Care Association
RHA Treasurers
Royal College of Midwives
Royal College of Nursing
Royal College of Obstetricians & Gynæcologists
Royal College of Physicians
Royal College of Psychiatrists
Royal College of Surgeons
Society of Chiropodists
Society of Radiographers
Solihull Area Dental Advisory Committee
Standing Conference of Representatives of Health Visitor Training
    Centres
Standing Dental Advisory Committee
Standing Medical Advisory Committee
Standing Nursing & Midwifery Advisory Committee
Standing Pharmaceutical Advisory Committee

OTHER ORGANISATIONS

Age Concern (England)

Association of British Adoption and Fostering Agencies
Association of Spina Bifida & Hydrocephalus
British Polio Fellowship
British Red Cross Society
Church of England Children's Society
Counsel & Care for the Elderly
COHSE
Elderly Invalids Fund
Family Welfare Association
Foundation for the Study of Infant Deaths
Health Education Council
Hertfordshire Council for Voluntary Service
Howard League for Penal Reform
King Edward's Hospital Fund for London
Labour Campaign for Mental Health
MIND
Multiple Sclerosis Society
NALGO
National Association of Citizens Advice Bureaux
National Association of Leagues of Hospital Friends
National Association for Maternal & Child Welfare
National Association for the Welfare of Children in Hospital
National Association of Voluntary Help Organisers
National Childbirth Trust
National Children's Bureau
National Council of Social Service
National Foster Care Association
National Training Council for the NHS
National Staff Committees
NATSOPA
NSPCC
Panel of Four (Associations for the Deaf)
Pre-School Playgroups Association
Public Health Laboratory Service Board
Royal National Institute for the Blind
Royal Society of Health
The Order of St. John
Social Welfare Commission
Soroptimist International
Southwark Trades Council
Spastics Society
Trades Union Congress
University of London
VOLCUF
Volunteer Centre
West of England Schizophrenia Society
Women's National Cancer Campaign
Women's Royal Voluntary Service

APPENDIX II

Summary of main points arising from analysis of RHA Strategic Plans

1 **General** The policies proposed in the consultative document were endorsed in principle: the main divergences arose from practical problems of implementation.

2 **Services for the mentally ill and mentally handicapped** All regions foresaw slow progress in providing district-based services for the mentally ill and handicapped and in closing large psychiatric hospitals. There were widespread doubts about the ability of local authorities, despite joint financing, to provide residential and day care services for these groups. Most regions still had large institutionalised populations. Several commented on the increased revenue cost of providing treatment in smaller centres. But the main problem appeared to be a conflict, at least in the shorter term, between the priority for services for the mentally ill and mentally handicapped proposed in the consultative document, and the pressures on regions to invest in acute services. The Thames regions maintained that they had to use capital first for rationalisation of acute services in Inner London and expansion, eg in Essex and Kent. Some above-target regions were already committed to major capital developments to remedy deficiencies in acute services and to expand medical teaching, which would use up a large proportion of both capital and additional revenue at the expense of other priority developments.

3 **Maternity Services and Acute Services** The need to rationalise maternity services, to take account of the fall in the birth rate, and to reduce acute services where these were over-provided was generally accepted. Many regions clearly faced difficulties in securing the scale of change required in the acute services. Most existing teaching hospitals were in inner-city areas which had been losing population for many years, and patients had therefore been drawn from surrounding areas to sustain an adequate work load. It seemed unlikely that, even in the long term, acute services, eg in the Thames regions, could be spread equitably without reducing teaching commitments in Inner London. Some regions suggested that redistribution of acute services and reduction of cross boundary patient flows should be a very low priority where the transport network was good enough to avoid serious inconvenience to patients.

4 **Population and resource assumptions** All regions were concerned about the uncertainty over future population assumptions, especially internal migration and the birth rate, and future levels of resources. Appendix V gives some additional guidance on future resource assumptions. In 1978 the OPCS are producing further guidance on population projections.

5 Manpower Planning It is too soon to expect manpower planning to have reached a high level, nationally or locally. Few plans presented a manpower strategy tailored to regional needs. Some regions made creditable attempts. Without a common format for plans it was difficult to bring together general staffing demand trends, though national policy was generally accepted. The major need was for more quantification, a closer relationship with financial forecasts and service proposals, better base line information and a greater appreciation of training requirements. Central and local manpower planning will require development before the next strategic plans are produced.

6 Planning Method Most plans contained a review of existing services, a statement of longer term objectives and of needs for service development and redistribution. Some plans did not deal with some important services which need to be covered. Most plans did not relate needs for service development to plans for the future development of resources including finance, manpower and physical assets. Closure programmes were not generally specified in any detail: such programmes are necessary for assessing priorities and the pace of change. Generally, there had not yet been time to link regional and area strategies or to assess how far operational plans would lead to implementation of strategies over the next 3 years.

More effective use of NHS resources: examples

1 The examples of possible ways of obtaining the more effective management of resources listed in this appendix have been touched on in discussions and meetings Ministers have held with staff groups in the NHS over the first half of 1977. In most cases the suggestions are based on studies and experiments in particular health authorities. Many authorities and their staffs therefore will know of these ideas, but it is hoped that bringing them together in one document will be helpful to everyone concerned with the use of resources.

2 The list is not comprehensive and authorities wanting more information are asked to contact the appropriate Regional Principal, RL Division, DHSS, Euston Tower, London NW1 3DN.

3 First, however, authorities may wish to be reminded of:

a. *Guide to Good Practices.* This was last published in 1970 and contains a considerable amount of information on the effective management of resources. A revised edition will be published later in 1977.

b. *Notes on Good Practices.* This new series is being launched in September 1977, and replaces the former series of *Abstracts of Efficiency.* The new series will repeat some of those abstracts that have been found to be particularly useful as well as producing new information. Some of the subjects in preparation are: community nursing, hospital admissions, pooling of beds, mobile chiropody service, school health records, and appointments procedures in health centres. These notes will be circulated to district management teams, clinicians, senior nursing staff and management services staff, and will form a major channel for the dissemination of information on good practices.

c. "Management Survey". This technique is designed to improve the effectiveness of the organisation and practices of a hospital (or of departments) by means of a rapid survey based on the results of past detailed studies. Experience has shown that the application of this technique can yield efficiency improvements of at least 5 per cent.

Authorities wanting more information on these items should contact D V Chislett, Central Management Services, DHSS, Ray House, 6 St Andrew Street, London EC4 3AD.

4 Medical and nursing

A number of suggestions for the more effective use of medical and nursing resources are listed at paragraphs A to E below: these are based on proven studies and procedures already obtaining in the Service, and may therefore be of general interest. First, however, there are two general points to be made:

a. The better (ie more intensive) use of a particular resource may lead to more patients being dealt with, so that the overall cost to an employing authority increases. The cost of treating the individual patient may fall, but with more patients being treated the total cost may rise. Some of the suggestions listed below will result in a higher patient throughput.

b. The following suggestions relate mainly to improvements of administrative arrangements, and *not* to specific clinical policies.

A **Hospital beds**
i. Major improvements have been achieved by the allocation of beds in the major specialty divisions into two blocks, dealing respectively with the *acute* and *elective* work in each major specialty grouping. The pooling of beds within these specialty groupings can lead to improved bed usage and greater ease in admitting acute emergencies. A telephone call-in procedure for patients requiring elective treatment gives time to call a second patient if one fails for any reason to be able to accept the bed. In situations where demand for beds far outstrips available resources the designation of a medically qualified admissions officer with full authority to decide on priorities has proved to be useful.

ii. The *length of stay* in many hospital units can be reduced by the timely and appropriate assistance of other specialists (eg geriatricians) and other health care professionals. Patterns of shared care such as an orthopaedic/geriatric unit are emerging which show not only benefit to the patient but also improved use of hospital beds.

iii. *Lengths of stay* for surgical patients have tended to be arbitrarily defined. The recent concept of "right stay" surgery matches the stay in hospital to what is clinically safe, appropriate in the eyes of the patient, family and general practitioner and yet is no longer than is necessary for a safe clinical recovery. [" 'Right' stay in hospital after surgery". Randomised controlled trial: Simpson, Cox, Meade, Brennan and Lee: *BMJ* 11 June 1977, p.1514.]

iv. Some patients needing elective surgical procedures may be safely selected for treatment in *day care units* or from *five day wards*. Such units can lead to a higher patient throughput and decreased nursing requirements outside normal working hours without detriment to patient care. The institution of such units has implications for anaesthetic care and some departments have set up anaesthetic clinics to assess patients pre-operatively.

v. Patients who require hospital admission for investigation either because of the complexity or the volume of investigations may best be admitted to a *Programmed Investigation Unit*. In such units patients are only admitted after all their investigations have been planned and booked. ["Programmed Investigation Units": Longson and Young: *BMJ* 1 December 1973.]

vi. Criteria for the admission and retention of patients in *intensive care units* should be reviewed, and adhered to, as excess capacity in them is expensive to maintain.

B   Operating theatres

Some authorities have found that the timetabling and allocation of theatre sessions in the week are not related to the pattern of work and other resources, ie hospital beds, and admitting procedures of different specialties. As with bed usage, experience shows that the effective organisation of operating theatres requires co-operation between surgeons, anaesthetists and nurses and information about how the resource has been used.

C   Radiology and pathology departments

With increasing demands on limited resources radiologists and pathologists should discuss with their clinical colleagues the most effective and economic use of these support services. A number of studies have now been completed which show that certain commonly ordered tests/examinations may be of little use in the management of particular patients. Control by consultants of the ordering habits of junior staff may significantly reduce the number of unnecessary and often costly investigations.

D   Out-patient departments

Among ideas which are worth considering are:—

i. Consultation time in out-patients will be more effective if as much information about patients has already been obtained from referral letters, and by the use of questionnaires completed by patients prior to appointments, and if essential tests have already been ordered. Not all of this appointment screening can be delegated to administrative staff.

ii. Long-term and unnecessary follow-up in out-patient departments may occur when junior staff are unsure whether or not to discharge a patient from hospital surveillance.

iii. Nurse staffing of out-patient clinics may be more effective, or savings achieved, if nurses are relieved of functions which do not require nursing skills.

iv. To enable general practitioners to obtain the best service for their patients, some hospitals periodically circularise all practitioners using their hospital with information about the waiting times for their clinics.

E   Primary health care

i. The time that community nursing staff spend on professional duties can be increased when general medical practitioners practice within defined geographical areas.

ii. The confidence of primary care teams in early discharge or return of patients to community care (saving hospital costs) depends on good and prompt communication from the hospital about individual patients. Studies (and individual complaints) still show that some hospitals take far too little trouble about this.

iii. The introduction of a community night nursing service allows patients who are terminally ill or who might otherwise require hospital beds to remain at home. Where such a service is operating, it might be hospital based in order fully to utilise the nursing time and improve communications.

5 DRUG PRESCRIBING

a. A number of hospitals have, after consultation among consultants and pharmacists, produced their own local formulary; only drugs on this list are kept in the pharmacy. The development of agreed prescribing policies can lead to major savings in hospital drug costs. Hospital-decided policies moreover will profoundly influence follow-up prescribing by general practitioners.

b. Some hospitals run "medical economy groups", covering drugs, equipment etc. It may be valuable to circulate information locally about comparative costs of drugs with identical properties to doctors and nurses, both in hospital and in general practice.

6. PROCUREMENT

a. The Secretary of State has already announced the setting up of a working group under the chairmanship of Mr Brian Salmon to consider the establishment of a Supply Board.

b. By pursuing the Department's recommended central stores policy, one area health authority has saved sufficient money in the first year of a partially centralised system of storage and distribution to fund a lease for accommodation to provide a completely centralised system (producing even more savings) and also to make available over £100,000 for direct patient care. These savings will be continuous and will accrue from the reduction in overall stores staffing levels within the area, use of mechanical handling and other stores aids, more efficient stock control and re-ordering methods and the facility to accept orders in large drops.

c. Central services can be helpful as a source of information for purchasing. If an item is already "approved" by the Department, it is a waste of money to inspect factories and examine samples.

d. "Cut down waste" campaigns in the use of dressings, bandages etc are worth considering, and might lead to substantial savings. Preferences for more expensive brands could be probed: in some cases a "butter or marge" type of test has demonstrated the irrationality of some preferences.

e. Greater use should be made of existing contracts placed by the Department and at regional and area levels. Time and effort spent in negotiating contracts for similar products at different levels due mainly to user prejudice is wasted.

7 BUILDING: SPACE UTILISATION

The capital value of existing NHS building stock in replacement terms is estimated to be about £7,000m. It is therefore important that the maximum use is made of this valuable asset. A more effective use of the space provided by building (perhaps by shared-use or multi-use of space) can:

help to improve patient throughput and reduce waiting lists;
lead to a more effective use of staff resources and save revenue;
reduce the requirement for new buildings and save capital;
make some existing buildings redundant, saving revenue and perhaps contributing to capital by their sale.

8 MAINTENANCE OF BUILDINGS, ENGINEERING PLANT AND GROUNDS

a. Preventing unnecessary deterioration by maintaining buildings at the correct time saves money. For instance if the external painting of wood windows is delayed for two years the subsequent remedial work will often double the cost of repainting. If the wood is neglected and allowed to rot away replacement may cost 5 times as much as regular painting. This can be applied to other kinds of building maintenance. Similarly, neglected engineering maintenance can result in costly repair bills, as well as creating the risk of breakdowns in essential services and serious hazards to patients and staff.

b. Using the most economical means of executing maintenance work and achieving maximum productivity will enable more work to be carried out for the same money. For example, studies have shown that it is possible to save up to 20 per cent of the cost by selecting the correct method of executing painting work, a type of work which accounts for over 10 per cent of total expenditure on maintenance.

c. One district has found it possible to save £21,000 pa on a budget of £63,000, ie 33 per cent, by adopting a more economical way of maintaining grounds and gardens.

d. Worthwhile savings can be made from a re-design of hospital grounds which keeps maintenance requirements to a minimum without losing desirable visual features for the amenity of patients and staff. Departmental guidance on grounds maintenance illustrates an example of a West Country hospital where annual maintenance costs were reduced to less than a quarter of previous levels and conversion costs recouped in the first year by rationalising the layout of grounds and by the elimination of many labour-intensive gardening activities.

e. The value of planning the maintenance programme and the need for continuous review of the time interval between planned and routine tasks is widely accepted, so there is a need to review critically the frequencies at which planned preventive maintenance and other routine tasks are carried out in order to optimise the cost-effectiveness of plant and equipment.

f. £30m is spent annually on contract maintenance. Some maintenance tasks are best executed by well trained and managed, directly employed

..men; in other cases greater use of term contractors is more economical. Each case needs to be assessed on its merits and it is wrong to stick to a single method.

g. Much damage to buildings could be avoided if all vehicles used in health buildings were adequately buffered.

9 CAPITAL EXPENDITURE

a. Cost limits prevent waste overall but a sensible distribution of expenditure within the limits is still required. Expensive materials and finishes which contribute nothing to function or to reducing maintenance are a poor bargain and should be avoided. Space standards as well as space utilisation should be critically examined.

b. For every £1,000 capital expenditure on engineering equipment and services another £1,000 will be needed for maintenance during its life. Requests for services requiring the provision of air conditioning plant, piped medical gas installations, call services, patient bed facilities and other engineering equipment should be critically examined and, where possible, less complex alternatives suggested.

c. **Nucleus hospital** The complete package for an initial range of departments will be available by the end of 1977. The use of standard design material offers a way of achieving the best use of scarce planning resources. It can also lead to savings to authorities of professional fees — guidance on this aspect will be issued shortly. Primarily intended to meet the need for a "hot core" acute hospital—initially of some 300 beds at a cost of £6m (1975 prices), but capable of expansion — the designs should also be considered for expansion and development schemes to maximise the integration and rationalisation of existing buildings and services. Briefing material and policies may be of value to authorities in their own design programmes. A few of the cost saving features of Nucleus are: planning of functional relationships to allow multi-use of space and sharing of facilities; maximum use of natural light and ventilation; restriction to a maximum of three storeys; a phasing and expansion strategy including planned alternative use of accommodation in the initial phases.

d. **Manufacturers Data Base (MDB) and Activity Data Base (ADB)** Use of the full health building system being developed to provide a systematic and co-ordinated method of carrying out all the operations involved throughout the process of a health building project is expected to yield very considerable savings. Two important parts of the system, ADB and MDB, have so far been made available to authorities and their use in appropriate circumstances can yield worthwhile savings.

10 LAND DISPOSAL

NHS land may well be worth more than £200m. Authorities should ensure that their property holdings do not exceed needs and take steps to dispose of any surpluses. For example three sales of land in 1976/77 brought in £500,000, £130,000 and £120,000.

11 ENERGY SAVING

The cost of energy consumption by the NHS in 1976/77 is estimated to have been about £130m. Energy saving can be an obvious contributor to the better use of NHS resources. Over the past four years 1973/74 to 1976/77, the NHS has achieved savings of just over 20 per cent in primary fuel consumption, ie an average of 5 per cent per annum, and a small saving in electricity consumption of about $4\frac{1}{2}$ per cent, when compared with what energy consumption would have been if the trend of the six years 1967/68 to 1972/73 had continued. These savings have been achieved through the implementation of small capital schemes to reduce the unnecessary consumption of energy such as by roof insulation and heating controls and by the co-operation of all staff in observing the basic principles of good housekeeping (switching off lights when not needed, avoiding overheating, turning down radiators rather than opening windows and closing down completely on heating and lighting facilities when departments are not in use overnight or at weekends). At current prices 1 per cent saving in primary fuel represents £950,000 per annum. And there is still scope for further savings. Staff should be asked to maintain and improve their response to the "save it" campaign. Authorities should review their building stock to consider whether there are areas which would benefit from small capital investment schemes with a short term (up to three years) pay-back from energy savings, and will continue to accrue to the benefit of the services when pay-back is completed. The benefit of the savings will increase in line with increases in the relative cost of energy; it has been estimated that the cost of energy will increase by 5 per cent per annum from 1980 to become double in real terms by the year 2000.

12 AMBULANCES

a. The pattern of ambulance (non-emergency) traffic should be reviewed and steps taken to use ambulances more efficiently by closer co-ordination between out-patient departments and ambulance controllers. The need for out-patients to travel by ambulance should be periodically reviewed.

b. Maintenance and supply aspects of all hospital transport should be examined, as these can be unnecessarily costly. One authority paid £80 each for flashing lights that were available at half the cost.

c. One region has already halved the number of ambulance controls and further reduction is planned, leading to a total saving of about £150,000 a year.

13 CATERING AND DOMESTIC SERVICES

Catering, domestic services and the linen and laundry services together cost the NHS about £535m a year. There is scope for substantial savings in this area, while maintaining standards.

a. Meal services for patients
i. Research has shown that bulk food trolley services are extremely wasteful and savings are possible by the introduction of a plated meal service. Although this type of service is not necessarily practical

in all hospitals or for the service to all patients, it is possible that the introduction of a simple plate service system requiring minimal capital expenditure would effect substantial savings in many hospitals.

ii. Authorities should ensure that efficient control and ordering systems are established for the direct issue of provisions to hospital wards. This is often a high cost area where savings may be made without reducing the standard of patient meals.

iii. There is evidence of extensive use of expensive proprietary products in feeding patients where less expensive foods are equally suitable. This is usually for convenience, or the lack of awareness of the alternative. Some of the products are very expensive and even a small usage can add up to a large cost.

iv. Where patients can choose dishes and portion size, less food is wasted. The need to offer three course meals and cooked breakfasts should be reviewed.

b. Authorities should explore the possibility of procuring more food items with long shelf life through the national contracting arrangements.

c. Food Waste.   Savings may be achieved by the identification of the extent and cause of food waste in hospitals to show how it could be avoided and to set targets for reducing it. One estimate of the extent of avoidable food waste — at £10 a day — would, if grossed up to national level, yield savings of £10m per year.

d. Bulk water boilers in kitchens when operated under properly controlled conditions (with thermostatic and "boost" controls) have been shown to use 60 per cent less fuel than when operated manually.

e. Health authorities should ensure that policies for domestic services are adequately considered and reviewed at high level, since this may throw up opportunities for rationalisation and economy. For example, perhaps more use would be made of the recently introduced grade of domestic ward orderly which embraces a wide range of tasks and might replace some outdated job structures. There may be duplication of management tasks between specialist domestic service managers and general administrators, and scope for the specialist skills to be applied more effectively over a wider range of the hospitals' "hotel services".

f. A number of hospitals have successfully introduced ward house-keeping or hotel schemes. The main duties from which nurses should be relieved are cleaning wards and annexes, washing up and general domestic work, and clerical tasks which take them from the bedside.

g. Sound cleaning techniques avoid expensive damage. One ruined operating theatre floor cost £60,000 to replace.

h. Laundry Services. Improved liaison between laundry and wards may help to cut down the amount of stocks of sheets etc required as well as the number of items sent for washing.

There may be scope for reducing the cost of laundry services. In one laundry the Secretary of State visited, unit costs were 30 per cent below the national average.

APPENDIX IV
Public expenditure decisions

England. £ million. 1976 Survey Prices

	1977/78	1978/79	1979/80
Hospital and Community Health			
Capital			
Cmnd 6393	284	284	284
Cmnd 6721	259	264	278
Current			
Cmnd 6393	3,242	3,283	3,326
Cmnd 6721	3,241[1]	3,281[1]	3,322[1]
Family Practitioner Services			
Current			
Cmnd 6393	953	981	1,011
Cmnd 6721	927	935	966
LA Personal Social Services			
Capital			
Cmnd 6393	47	47	47
Cmnd 6721	39	39	39
Current			
Cmnd 6393	780	796	812
Cmnd 6721	786	802	821
Centrally Financed Services[2]			
Capital			
Cmnd 6393	13	12	9
Cmnd 6721	8	11	10
Current			
Cmnd 6393	202	200	198
Cmnd 6721	200[3]	200	199
Totals			
Cmnd 6393	5,521	5,603	5,687
Cmnd 6721	5,461	5,533	5,635

NB Discrepancies in totals are due to rounding.
[1] Includes addition to take account of loss of revenue growing out of withdrawal of proposed road traffic legislation.
[2] Includes other health services, Central Government PSS, and Central Miscellaneous Services.
[3] Excludes savings of £1·5m made to offset addition in note (1).

APPENDIX V

Resource allocations to RHAs

1 Planning Guidelines issued to the NHS in May 1977 (HC(77)19) based on the latest Public Expenditure White Paper (Cmnd 6721), gave regional resource assumptions for planning for the period to 1979/80 and said that:

For the period beyond 1979/80 RHAs should assume *for planning purposes only*

a. a revenue growth rate nationally similar to that assumed for 1978/79 and 1979/80, and a similar basis of allocation between regions;

b. capital resources nationally remaining at about the level indicated for 1978/79 and 1979/80.

Both revenue and capital planning should be sufficiently flexible to take account of the possibility of significant variations either way.

2 An analysis taking account of those factors affecting resource allocation which are more readily susceptible of prediction suggests that on the long-term national resource assumptions described above the *average annual growth* in revenue allocations (excluding SIFT and joint finance) received by each RHA, other than the Thames regions, over the period from the 1977/78 base to 1986/87 would be of broadly the following proportions:

Northern	2·0%	Oxford	1·3%
Yorkshire	1·5%	South Western	1·9%
Trent	2·4%	West Midlands	1·9%
East Anglian	2·4%	Mersey	1·2%
Wessex	2·4%	North Western	2·0%

3 For the Thames regions, the statement of the Secretary of State on 21 December 1976 on the RAWP Report announced a growth rate of 0·25 per cent for the best-provided Thames regions and somewhat higher increases for the other Thames regions; and the DHSS planning guidelines for 1977/78 (HC(77)19) assumed no growth in these regions for 1978/79 and 1979/80, and the continuation of similar assumptions for the years beyond 1979/80. This document does not change these assumptions.

4 Significant variations in resource assumptions to be allowed for in planning might reasonably cover a range of ±50 per cent of the average annual rates of addition in para 2. For the Thames regions, variation for planning purposes might include the possibility of a small average annual reduction or a modest annual addition (accruing mainly in the later years) of 0·2 per cent for NW, NE and SE Thames, and up to 0.6 per cent for SW Thames. RHAs will be able to foresee the probable pattern of additions over the period assumed in this forecast starting from their 1977/78 rate of addition and falling, rising or remaining relatively stable.

5   Comparison of the figures in Table 1 attached to HC(77)19 for 1978/79 and 1979/80 indicates the general level and direction of increase or decrease of capital allocations in the early years of the decade ahead. The figures are affected by known commitments but, for the period up to 1985/86, RHAs should plan for significant variations on either side of the 1979/80 figure.

APPENDIX VI

The 1977 programme budget : Background note

1 A full description of the purpose and methodology of the programme budget is given in Annex 2 to the consultative document (CD). This note describes certain features of the 1977 programme budget, which forms the basis of figures 2-5 and takes account of the actual position in 1975/76 as well as comments made on the CD.

The 1975/76 base
2 The out-turn figures from the accounts and costing returns were adjusted in accordance with the public expenditure survey costing conventions and analysed essentially by the same method as last year. However, because the 1977 programme budget is based on the new NHS accounting returns, there are some technical changes compared with the format in the CD. The main change is that administrative costs are identified separately instead of being included in expenditure on particular services. Allowing for this, the out-turn of expenditure on hospital services in 1975/76 was fairly close to the provisional estimate in the CD except that expenditure on acute services was somewhat higher, and on geriatrics somewhat lower, than estimated.

3 Similarly, administrative costs are now identified separately in the analysis of LA expenditure on the personal social services; there is no longer separate provision for "training", and intermediate treatment is shown separately instead of being included in "other LA services". The actual unit costs of residential places for children (including mentally handicapped children) proved to be higher than estimated in the CD but those for the mentally ill were lower; costs of places in day nurseries were also considerably higher than estimated.

Projections to 1979/80
4 The projections for 1979/80 in figures 3 to 5 provide a quantitative assessment of national priorities at a level of expenditure compatible with the plans set out in Cmnd 6721. As in the CD, *the figures are purely illustrative.*

5 The projections are based upon the analysis of out-turn expenditure in 1975/76 and estimates of future growth. In some instances, eg family practitioner services, the 1979/80 figures represent a forecast of expected demand. For other services, to start with estimates were made of the potential cost of developments taking account of past trends in activity and unit costs, demographic change, specific policies for various client groups, the effect of recent legislation and general priorities. The resulting figure for total potential expenditure was then compared with the level of

46

public expenditure planned in Cmnd 6721 for the health and personal social services, and the proposals for development of the various services adjusted so as to bring the total projected expenditure to that level.

6   Unit costs in both health and personal social services are generally assumed to be higher than in the CD projections, to allow for expenditure on such items as fire precautions, and health and safety at work. However, for obstetrics, the total projected expenditure is slightly reduced though, with fewer forecast births, the cost per in-patient case is not reduced as much as suggested in the CD.

NOTES ON FIGURES 2-5
Common detail
7   (a) All figures are approximate and discrepancies are due to rounding. Levels of provision and expenditure per head less than unity are shown to 2 decimal places to illustrate the trends between 1975/76 and 1979/80: this does not imply greater accuracy than for quantities quoted to one decimal place.

(b) The 1976 based population projections are used throughout.

Figure 2
8   To assist in the analysis of plans, DHSS has completed from centrally available statistics and costing returns a standard check list of information about each region in 1975/76.

Figure 2 sets out current expenditure per head on programmes as defined for the national programme budget but covering Health and Community Health Services only and excluding Service Increment for Teaching (SIFT) and preserved BG expenditure. These figures give only a crude comparison and should be treated with caution:

(a) the population denominators (often "whole population") are not weighted by age or SMRs;

(b) they disguise considerable internal variation, eg in NE Thames an above target area spent twice as much per head as a below target area.

In addition, mental handicap and mental illness figures have not been adjusted to take account of institutional populations.

9   Regional comparisons should take account of the different age structure, mortality etc of different regions. The final column takes account of weighting by measures of relative health care need and adjustments for cross-boundary flows.

Figure 3
10   The CD provisional estimate for 1975/76 shown in Figure 3 differs from that in the CD because of the following changes:

(a) as described in paragraph 2, administration is now separately identified and here mostly included under "other services";

(b) "other services" also includes SIFT;

(c) "clinics" have been transferred from children's services to primary care.

11 As regards the 1979/80 projections:

(a) compared with 1975/76 the primary care share increases by 1% instead of by 1·6% as shown in the CD because increased charges and proposed drug economies will reduce gross expenditure;

(b) LA capital on services for the elderly and younger physically handicapped is much lower, partly offsetting the rise in current expenditure;

(c) current expenditure on children's services rises faster, because of increasing unit costs of residential care.

12 The various expenditure blocks are made up as follows:

(a) general and acute hospital and maternity services:
  —Acute IP & OP
  —Ambulances
  —SIFT
  —Other hospital (blood transfusion service etc)
  —Obstetric IP & OP
  —Midwives.

(b) primary care:
  —Family Practitioner Services
  —Prevention
  —Family Planning
  —Other Community Health.

(c) services mainly for the elderly or physically handicapped:
  —Geriatric IP & OP
  —Non-psychiatric DP
  —Home nursing
  —Chiropody
  —Residential care
  —Home Help
  —Meals
  —Day Care
  —Aids, adaptations, phones etc
  —Services for the disabled.

(d) other services:
  —Social work
  —Other LA services
  —Hospital and Community Health Administration
  —LA administration
  —Miscellaneous Centrally Financed Services.

(e) services for the mentally ill:
  —Mental Illness IP & OP

—Psychiatric DP
—Residential care
—Day care
—Special hospitals.

(f) services mainly for children:
—Health visiting
—School health
—Residential care
—Welfare food
—Boarding out
—Day nurseries
—Intermediate treatment
—Central grants and Youth Treatment Centres.

(g) services for the mentally handicapped:
—Mental Handicap IP & OP
—Residential Care
—Day Care.

Figure 4

13 (a) The acute inpatient guideline relates to new hospitals.

(b) "Other hospital" includes SIFT, mass radiography, blood transfusion service, income and accounting adjustments.

(c) The category "non-psychiatric day patients" covers attendances by geriatric patients and also other patients, eg in units for the younger disabled or those needing intermittent dialysis. The guideline of 2·7 places per 1,000 population aged 65 years and over is made up of 2·0 places for geriatric patients and 0·7 places for other patients.

(d) "Other Community Health" includes clinics, health centres, etc.

(e) The cost per place for non-psychiatric and mental illness day patients is based on an assumption of 200 attendances per place.

Figure 5

14 (a) The levels of provision for the elderly and younger disabled include accommodation in voluntary and private homes — 19,000 places and 4,000 places respectively.

(b) "Social Workers" includes social work assistants and trainees.

APPENDIX VII
BIBLIOGRAPHY

I Main source documents on good practices

a. Management Services (NHS) No. 1 — Guide to Good Practices in Hospital Administration (HMSO 1970) (Revision in preparation).

b. DHSS, Central Management Services, List of Recent Publications (DHSS).

c. Estmancode—Estate Management (Building, Engineering and Grounds) Practices Code for the NHS (DHSS and Welsh Office).

d. Abstracts of Efficiency Studies in the NHS (the title of this series has recently been changed to Notes on Good Practices) (HMSO).

f. Management Services (NHS) Reports (HMSO).

II Selected references

Management Services (NHS) Reports
- No. 2 —Work of nurses in out-patient departments.
- No. 5 —Work measurement in radio-diagnostic departments.
- No. 6 —Organisation and management of hospital linen services.
- No. 7 —Study of work in hospital kitchens to determine staffing ratios

Hospital O & M Service Reports
- No. 1 —Out-patient Waiting Time.
- No. 2 —Medical Records and Secretarial Services.
- No. 6 —Pathology—measurement of work in units.
- No. 9 —Ordering and receipt of pharmaceutical supplies.

Hospital O & M and Work Study Reports
- No. 11 —Hospital Portering Services.
- No. 12 —Organisation and Management of Hospital Laundries.

Abstracts of Efficiency Studies in the NHS/Notes on Good Practices
- No. 140—Cardio-vascular Department—use of ECG machine.
- No. 167—ENT Department—Increasing bed occupancy.
- No. 168—Catering—Control of Food Costs.
- No. 171—Nursing—the most time consuming activities of nurses in geriatric wards.
- No. 174—Programmed Investigation Bed.
- No. 175—Programmed Investigation and Treatment Unit.
- No. 179—One Day Minor Surgery Unit.

Hospital Building Notes
- No. 6 —Diagnostic X-ray Departments.

NCB ORE Reports — issued by DHSS
- Centralisation of stores.
- Stock control systems in hospital stores.

Other reports and publications.
    Interim Report of Steering Committee on standardisation of supplies
    from CSSDs (DHSS).
    The Standardisation of Hospital Medical Records.
    Report of the Specification Working Party on Office Area Furniture
    (DHSS).
    Management Services Handbook — Typing Services (Civil Service
    Department).

III Additions to the Consultative Document list of published reports on innovation in clinical practice

Value of new laboratory tests in diagnosis and treatment (W W Holland
and T P Whitehead, *Lancet* (August 17) *2*, 391, 1974).

Making do: Chemical-pathology services (M G Rinsler, *Lancet* (April 30)
1, 946, 1977).

The preoperative chest X-ray, a study of its over-use in non-cardio-
pulmonary surgery (A M Rees, C J Roberts, A S Bligh, C T Evans,
BMJ, 1, 1333, 1976).

Radiology now, The Radiologist's Dilemma, (C T Evans, *British Journal
of Radiology, 50*, 299, 1977).

IV List of documents referred to in the main text

Allen, I., 1976. *Family planning services in the home.* (Broadsheet No. 565)
London, Political and Economic Planning.

Department of the Environment. DoE Circular 120/76: LAC(76)28. *Rate
support grant settlement 1977/78.*

Department of the Environment, Scottish Home and Health Department
and Welsh Office, 1977. *Policy for the inner cities* (Cmnd 6845) London,
HMSO.

Department of Health and Social Security (RHB Chairmen 10/69).
Interim measures to improve hospital services for the mentally handicapped.

Department of Health and Social Security (RHB Chairmen 10/70).
Services for the mentally handicapped.

Department of Health and Social Security and Welsh Office, 1971.
Better services for the mentally handicapped. (Cmnd 4683) London,
HMSO.

Department of Health and Social Security (HSC(IS)75). *National Health
Service: development of health services: community hospitals.*

Department of Health and Social Security (HSC(IS)181). *Reduction of
waiting times for in-patients admission: management arrangements.*

Department of Health and Social Security, 1976. *Prevention and health:
everybody's business: a reassessment of public and personal health.* London,
HMSO.

Department of Health and Social Security, 1976. *Sharing resources for
health in England: report of the Resource Allocation Working Party.*
London, HMSO.

Department of Health and Social Security (HC(77)17) (LAC(77)10). *Joint care planning: health and local authorities.*

Expenditure Committee. Session 1976-77. *First report . . . together with the minutes of evidence taken before the Social Services and Employment Sub-Committee in Sessions 1975-76 and 1976-77, appendices and index: preventive medicine.* 3 vols. (HC 169-i, ii and iii) London, HMSO.

Joint Committee on Vaccination and Immunisation. 1977. *Whooping cough vaccination: Review of the evidence on whooping cough vaccination by the Joint Committee on Vaccination and Immunisation.* London, HMSO.

Treasury, 1976. *Public expenditure to 1979-80.* (Cmnd 6393) London, HMSO.

Treasury, 1977. *The Government's expenditure plans.* (Cmnd 6721) 2 vols, London, HMSO.

Printed in England for Her Majesty's Stationery Office by Oyez Press Limited
Dd 586516 K280 8/77